I0790670

Table of Contents

Aging is a gradual, continuous process of natural change that begins in early adulthood. During early middle age, many bodily functions begin to gradually decline.

People do not become old or elderly at any specific age. Traditionally, age 65 has been designated as the beginning of old age. But the reason was based in history, not biology. Many years ago, age 65 was chosen as the age for retirement in Germany, the first nation to establish a retirement program. In 1965 in the United States, age 65 was designated as the eligibility age for Medicare insurance. This age is close to the actual retirement age of most people in economically advanced societies.

When a person becomes old can be answered in different ways:

Chronologic age is based solely on the passage of time. It is a person's age in years. Chronologic age has limited significance in terms of health. Nonetheless, the likelihood of developing a health problem increases as people age, and it is health problems, rather than normal aging, that are the primary cause of functional loss during old age. Because chronologic age helps predict many health problems, it has some legal and financial uses.

Biologic age refers to changes in the body that commonly occur as people age. Because these changes affect some people sooner than others, some people are biologically old at 65, and others not until a decade or more later. However, most noticeable differences in apparent age among people of similar chronologic age are caused by lifestyle, habit, and subtle effects of disease rather than by differences in actual aging.

Psychologic age is based on how people act and feel. For example, an 80-year-old who works, plans, looks forward to future events, and participates in many activities is considered psychologically younger.

Most healthy and active people do not need the expertise of a geriatrician (a doctor who specializes in the care of older people) until they are 70, 75, or even 80 years old. However, some people need to see a geriatrician at a younger chronologic age because of their medical conditions.

BREAKFAST

1. Corn and Bacon Frittata with Jalapeno

Prep Time: 10 Minutes

Cook Time: 35 Minutes

Servings: 4

Ingredients

- 3 slices center cut bacon, coarsely chopped
- 1/2 cup red onion, chopped finely
- 1 ear corn, cut off the cob
- 1 jalapeno, minced (or more)
- 8 eggs
- 1/4 cup skim milk
- 1/2 tsp Worcestershire sauce
- Salt and pepper

Instructions

1. Preheat the oven to 400 degrees. Cook the bacon in an oven-safe skillet until it is crispy.
2. Bacon cooking in a skillet.
3. Add the red onion and jalapeno and cook for about 6-8 minutes until the onion begins to be translucent.
4. Bacon, jalapenos, and red onion cooking in a skillet.
5. Add the corn and cook until cooked just through, about 3 minutes.

6. Corn, bacon, onions, and jalapenos cooking in a skillet.
7. Meanwhile, whisk together the eggs, egg whites, and milk. Stir in the salt, pepper, and Worcestershire sauce.
8. Eggs being whisked in a bowl.
9. Pour the egg mixture into the skillet.
10. Eggs being adding to a corn and bacon frittata.
11. Place the skillet in the oven and cook for an additional 20-25 minutes until the top is cooked through and the top gets slightly crispy.

Prep Time: 5 Minutes

Cook Time: 15 Minutes

Servings: 2

Ingredients

- 4 slices turkey bacon, chopped
- 3/4 cup shredded hash brown potatoes
- 2 green onions, chopped
- 4 eggs, whisked
- 4 corn tortillas
- Salt and pepper
- 1/4 cup salsa

Instructions

1. Heat a nonstick skillet over medium high heat. Add the bacon and cook for 2-3 minutes until beginning to get crispy.
2. Chopped turkey bacon cooking in a skillet.
3. Add the potatoes and green onions. Cook for 3-4 minutes until they begin to crisp.
4. Hash browns, green onions, and turkey bacon cooking in a skillet.
5. Push the potatoes, bacon, and green onions to one side of the pan. Spray with cooking spray and add the eggs. Let cook for a couple of minutes and then begin to scramble with the potatoes, bacon, and green onions. Cook to your liking.

6. Eggs cooking with hash browns, green onions, and
    bacon for tacos.
7. Warm the corn tortillas. Serve with the eggs and all
    your favorite toppings.

Prep Time: 15 Minutes

Cook Time: 30 Minutes

Servings: 4

Ingredients

- 1 lb. lean ground turkey sausage
- 2 tsp. olive oil
- 2 cups butternut squash, peeled and diced
- 1/2 red onion, diced
- 1/2 tsp. salt
- 1/2 tsp. garlic powder
- 1/2 tsp. oregano
- 1/2 tsp. pepper
- 4 cups spinach, chopped
- 4 eggs
- 4 egg whites

Instructions

1. Preheat the oven to 400 degrees. Heat a skillet over medium high heat. Add the sausage and cook until no longer pink, breaking it up as it cooks. Remove and set aside.
2. Ground turkey sausage browning in a skillet.
3. Add the olive oil to the pan. Once hot, add the butternut squash and red onion. Cook for 8-10 minutes until squash and onion are tender, adding 1-2 tablespoons of water if burning. Add the salt, garlic

powder, oregano, and pepper. Stir together. Add the
spinach and cook until it wilts, about 1-2 minutes.

4. Butternut squash, spinach, and red onion cooking in a
    skillet.
5. Whisk together the eggs. Add the sausage and
    butternut squash mixture to a baking dish sprayed
    with cooking spray. Pour the eggs over top.
6. Eggs being whisked in a bowl.
7. Bake for 25-30 minutes until eggs set and are cooked
    through.

Prep Time: 15 Minutes

Cook Time: 20 Minutes

Servings: 4

Ingredients

- 8 eggs
- 1/4 cup skim milk
- Salt and pepper
- 1/2 tbsp. olive oil
- 1/2 cup red onion, diced
- 1/2 cup green pepper, diced
- 1/2 cup red pepper, diced
- 1 cup diced lean ham
- 1 garlic clove, minced
- 1/2 cup shredded reduced fat cheddar cheese

Instructions

1. Preheat the broiler. Whisk together the eggs, egg whites, milk, salt, and pepper.
2. Eggs, milk, salt, and pepper being whisked in a bowl.
3. Heat the oil over medium heat in a nonstick pan. Add the onions, green peppers, and red peppers. Cook for 5-7 minutes until soft. Add the ham and garlic and cook for 2 minutes.
4. Diced ham, bell peppers, onions, and garlic cooking in a cast iron skillet.

5. Pour the egg mixture over the top and sprinkle cheese over top. Cook until edges are set and middle is just beginning to firm up, about 4-5 minutes.
6. Whisked eggs and shredded cheese being added to a skillet.
7. Place under the broiler, about 6 inches away, and cook until eggs are cooked through and puffed up about 3 minutes. Let cool and cut into slices to serve.
8. Western omelet frittata cit into slices and being served.

Prep Time: 10 Minutes

Cook Time: 25 Minutes

Servings: 8

Ingredients

- 1/2 tbsp olive oil
- 1/2 lb asparagus
- 1/4 chopped red onion
- 1 garlic clove, minced
- 6 eggs
- 1 cup nonfat milk
- 3/4 cup shredded part skim mozzarella cheese
- 1/4 cup crumbled feta cheese
- Salt and pepper to taste
- 1 refrigerated pie crust

Instructions

1. Preheat the oven to 375 degrees and place the frozen pie crust on the counter. In a large mixing bowl, whisk together the eggs. mozzarella and feta cheese, milk, salt, and pepper.
2. Eggs, milk, mozzarella cheese, feta cheese being whisked in a bowl.
3. Heat the olive oil in a skillet over medium high heat. Add the onions until they begin to become translucent. Add the asparagus and saute for 4-6 minutes until tender crisp. Add the garlic and cook for one minute until fragrant. Remove from heat.

4. Asparagus and red onion cooking in olive oil in a skillet.
5. Place the asparagus and onions in the bottom of the pie crust.
6. Asparagus spears in a unbaked pie crust.
7. Pour egg mixture on top. Bake for 35-40 minutes until the center is firm and no longer jiggles. Let cool at least 10 minutes.
8. Egg custard poured over asparagus spears in a pie crust.

Prep Time: 5 Minutes

Cook Time: 35 Minutes

Servings: 6

Ingredients

- 2 ripe bananas, mashed
- 1.5 cups unsweetened almond milk
- 1/4 cup unsweetened applesauce
- 2 tbsp brown sugar
- 1 egg
- 1 tsp cinnamon
- 1 tsp vanilla extract
- 1.5 cups old-fashioned oats
- 1/2 tsp baking powder
- 1/4 tsp salt

Instructions

1. Preheat the oven to 375 degrees. Spray an 8 by 8 pan with cooking spray or cover with parchment paper. Mash the bananas using a fork in a large bowl.
2. Add the milk, applesauce, brown sugar, and egg. Stir to combine.
3. Stir in the rolled oats, baking powder, and salt. Mix until just combined. If you are adding any extra ingredients, fold them into the oats here.
4. Pour into the baking dish. If desired, add a sprinkle of brown sugar over the top.

5. Bake for 35-40 minutes until golden brown. Let cool for 10-15 minutes before slicing.

Prep Time: 10 Minutes

Cook Time: 40 Minutes

Servings: 6

Ingredients

- 2 cups oats
- 1 tsp cinnamon
- 1/2 tsp salt
- 3/4 tsp baking powder
- 1.5 cups unsweetened apple sauce
- 1 cup unsweetened almond milk (or skim)
- 2 large eggs
- 2 tbsp. brown sugar
- 2 tbsp. maple syrup
- 1/2 tsp vanilla extract
- 1 cup fresh cranberries
- 1 apple, diced

Instructions

1. Preheat the oven to 375 degrees. Mix together the oats, salt, baking powder, and cinnamon. In another bowl, stir together the applesauce, almond milk, eggs, brown sugar, maple syrup, and vanilla extract.
2. Combine the dry and wet ingredients. Fold in the cranberries and apples. Pour into a baking dish (I used a 9 X 9 dish for 6 servings) sprayed with cooking spray.

3. Bake for 45 minutes until the oatmeal is golden brown and a toothpick comes out clean from the center. Let cool slightly and serve.

Prep Time: 15 Minutes

Cook Time: 50 Minutes

Servings: 6

Ingredients

- 1 lb apples, chopped
- 1/4 cup brown sugar (or honey/maple syrup)
- 1.5 tsp cinnamon
- 2 cups rolled oats
- 1/3 cup chopped walnuts (optional)
- 2 cups almond milk (or milk of choice)
- 1 egg
- 1 tsp vanilla extract
- 1 tsp baking powder
- 1/2 tsp salt

Instructions

1. Preheat the oven to 350 degrees. Spray an 8 X 8 baking dish with cooking spray. Add the apples to the baking dish. Toss with brown sugar and cinnamon. Cover with foil. Bake for 20 minutes.
2. Chopped apples in a baking dish being sprinkled with brown sugar.
3. Whisk together the milk, eggs, vanilla extract, baking soda, and salt in a large bowl. Stir in the oats and walnuts if using.
4. Rolled oats, walnuts, milk, and spices in a bowl.

5. Remove the apples from the oven carefully. Pour in the oatmeal mixture and stir to combine. Return to the oven uncovered.
6. Oatmeal being stirred into a baking dish with apples.
7. Bake for 30 minutes or until golden brown and set. Let rest for 10 minutes before cutting into slices.

Prep Time: 15 Minutes

Cook Time: 7hrs 50 Minutes

Servings: 6

Ingredients

- 1.5 cups dry steel cut oats
- 2 tbsp chia seeds
- 2 tbsp flaxseed meal
- 3 cups unsweetened vanilla almond milk
- 2 cups water
- 14 oz. canned pumpkin puree
- 3 tbsp pure maple syrup (more to taste)
- 1 tbsp pumpkin pie spice
- 1 tsp vanilla extract
- 1/2 tsp cinnamon
- 1/4 tsp salt

Instructions

1. Spray the slow cooker with cooking spray to prevent sticking. Add all the ingredients to the slow cooker and stir together.
2. Steel cut oats, almond milk, canned pumpkin, spices, chia seeds, and flaxseeds being stirred in a slow cooker.
3. Turn the slow cooker on low for 8 hours or high for 3.5-4 hours. This works great as an overnight recipe, put it in before you go to sleep and enjoy in the morning. I usually put this on right before I go to bed

because if it cooks too long it can get mushy. In the morning, you will wake up to delicious pumpkin pie oatmeal. This recipe will keep well in the fridge. I put mine in 1 cup servings and then just throw them in the microwave for a minute and they are ready to go. Add a little milk if needed when reheating.

Prep Time: 10 Minutes

Cook Time: 35 Minutes

Servings: 6

Ingredients

- 2 cups rolled oats
- 2 tbsp flaxseed meal
- 1 tsp cinnamon
- 1 tsp baking powder
- 1/2 tsp salt
- 2 cups unsweetened almond milk (or skim)
- 2 ripe bananas, mashed
- 3 tbsp pure maple syrup
- 1 tsp vanilla extract
- 1 egg

Instructions

1. Preheat the oven to 375 degrees. Spray an 8 X 8 baking sheet with cooking spray. In a large bowl, mix together the oats, flaxseed meal, cinnamon, baking powder, and salt.
2. Rolled oats, flaxseed meal, cinnamon, baking powder, and salt in a bowl.
3. In another bowl, mix together the milk, bananas, egg, maple syrup, and vanilla extract.
4. Milk, eggs, bananas, and maple syrup being stirred in a bowl.

5. Add the wet ingredients to the dry ingredients and stir until combined.
6. Rolled oats being combined with milk, bananas, and eggs in a bowl.
7. Pour into the baking dish. Bake for 35-40 minutes until cooked through and lightly browned on top.
8. Oatmeal being poured into a baking dish.
9. Top with fresh fruit, nuts, and/or maple syrup.

11. Zucchini and Ground Turkey Pizza Boats

Prep Time: 15 Minutes

Cook Time: 30 Minutes

Servings: 4

Ingredients

- 4 zucchini
- 1 tsp. olive oil
- 1/2 lb. 99% lean ground turkey
- 1 cup mushrooms, diced
- 2 garlic clove, minced
- 1/2 tsp. oregano
- 1/2 tsp. basil
- 1 cup marinara sauce
- 4 tbsp. Parmesan cheese
- 8 tbsp. part skim shredded mozzarella cheese

Instructions

1. Preheat the oven to 400 degrees.
2. Heat the olive oil over medium high heat. Add the turkey, mushrooms, and garlic. Cook until turkey is fully browned, about 6-8 minutes. Season with salt and pepper.
3. Stir in the oregano, basil, and marinara sauce.
4. Meanwhile cut the zucchini in half and scoop out some of the center using a spoon or melon baller to

create the "boat." Place in a baking dish sprayed with
cooking spray.
5. Fill the boats with the turkey and mushroom mixture.
6. Top each with 1 tbsp. of shredded cheese and 1/2 tbsp.
Parmesan cheese.
7. Bake for 15-18 minutes until cheese is bubbling and
zucchini is tender

Prep Time: 5 Minutes

Cook Time: 30 Minutes

Servings: 4

Ingredients

- 1 butternut squash
- 2 tbsp olive oil (for dressing)
- 6 cups arugula
- 1/3 cup almonds (roasted)
- 4 oz feta cheese, crumbled
- 3 tbsp fresh orange juice
- 1 tbsp red wine vinegar
- 1 tbsp honey
- 1/2 tsp kosher salt (more to taste)
- 1/4 tsp ground pepper (more to taste)

Instructions

1. Preheat the oven to 400 degrees. Cover a baking sheet with parchment paper or spray with cooking spray. Peel the butternut squash and chop into bite-sized pieces. Toss with olive oil, kosher salt, and pepper.
2. Roast the squash for 20 minutes until the bottoms begin to brown and caramelize. Shake the baking sheet, flipping the squash, and roast for 8-12 minutes until fork tender and lightly browned.
3. Meanwhile, whisk together the orange juice, olive oil, red wine vinegar, honey, salt, and pepper to make the dressing.

4. Assemble the salads with arugula, roasted butternut squash, feta cheese, almonds, and dressing.
5. For extra flavor, roast raw almonds. Preheat the oven to 350 degrees. Toss the almonds with olive oil, salt, pepper, and any herbs you like. Roast for 10-15 minutes until they are browned but not burnt.
6. This salad is delicious with fruit! Consider adding pomegranate seeds, dried cranberries, chopped apples, chopped pears, or dates.

Prep Time: 5 Minutes

Cook Time: 15 Minutes

Servings: 4

Ingredients

- 1 tbsp sesame oil (or olive)
- 1/2 red onion, diced
- 2 garlic cloves, minced
- 1 tbsp ginger, minced
- 1 lb. lean ground chicken (99% lean)
- 6 cups coleslaw mix
- 3/4 cup shelled edamame (leave out for Whole30)
- 4 tbsp reduced sodium soy sauce (or coconut aminos)
- 1 tbsp rice vinegar
- 2 tsp Sriracha (optional)
- 1/2 tsp black pepper

Instructions

1. Heat the sesame oil over medium high heat. Add the onion and cook 3-4 minutes. Add the garlic and ginger and cook for 1 minute until fragrant.
2. Red onion, garlic, and ginger in a skillet.
3. Add the chicken and cook, breaking it up with a wooden spoon, for 5-6 minutes until no longer pink.
4. Ground chicken cooking in a skillet with onions, garlic, and ginger.
5. Add the cole slaw mix and edamame. Stir. Mix together the soy sauce, rice vinegar, black pepper, and

Sriracha if using. Add to the pan and cook for 3-4 minutes until cabbage is tender-crisp. Taste and season with additional soy sauce if needed.

6. Ground chicken, cabbage, carrots, edamame, and soy sauce cooking in a skillet.

Prep Time: 5 Minutes

Cook Time: 25 Minutes

Servings: 4

Ingredients

- 1 tbsp olive oil
- 1 red onion, sliced thin
- 1 lb. shredded hash brown potatoes
- 2 garlic cloves, minced
- 1/4 tsp. red pepper flakes (optional)
- 1 zucchini, diced
- 1 red pepper, diced
- 2 cups broccoli florets (small florets)
- 1 cup mushrooms, sliced
- Salt and pepper
- 1 cup crumbled feta cheese

Instructions

1. Heat half the olive oil in a skillet over medium-high heat. Add the onions and let cook for 7-10 minutes until softened and just beginning to caramelize. Season with salt and pepper. Add the hash browns and stir to combine with the onions. Press down into the pan and let them crisp up on the bottom, cooking them for 3-4 minutes without moving them. Stir and repeat to get nice and crispy potatoes. Remove from the pan and set aside.

2. Hash brown potatoes being added to a skillet with red onions.

3. Add the remaining olive oil to the skillet with the garlic and red pepper flakes. Cook for 1 minute. Add the zucchini, red pepper, broccoli, and mushrooms. Cook for 7-10 minutes until tender-crisp, adding couple of tablespoons of water to the pan if the vegetables begin to burn. During this stage, cook the veggies to your desired tenderness. I prefer them to have some crunch still but you can cook them longer as well.

4. Fresh vegetables being stirred in a cast iron skillet.

5. Add the hash brown potatoes and onions back to the skillet and toss everything together. Cook for 1-2 minutes and season with salt and pepper. Serve with feta cheese on top. Many people eat this as a breakfast hash with eggs and toast but it also works great for lunch or dinner.

6. Hash browns and vegetables in a cast iron skillet with feta cheese crumbles.

Prep Time: 5 Minutes

Cook Time: 50 Minutes

Servings: 4

Ingredients

- 3 lbs. roma tomatoes, halved (or any mixture, ripe)
- 1 yellow onion, cut into quarters
- 8 garlic cloves (whole)
- 2 carrots, chopped (peeled)
- 1 red bell pepper, chopped
- 3 tbsp olive oil
- Salt and pepper
- 4 cups vegetable broth
- 1 tbsp balsamic vinegar
- 3 tbsp pesto

Instructions

1. Preheat the oven to 400 degrees. Add the tomatoes, onion, whole garlic cloves, carrots, and red pepper to a baking dish, Drizzle with olive oil and season well with salt and pepper.
2. Tomatoes, carrots, onion, and garlic on a baking sheet.
3. Roast for 45 minutes until the vegetables are tender, stirring the vegetables about halfway through cooking.
4. Roasted tomatos, onions, carrots, and garlic.
5. Add the roasted vegetables (and all the juice) to a large soup pot with the vegetable broth. Bring to a

simmer and then use a hand blender to puree until smooth.

6. Vegetable broth being added to a pot of roasted vegetables.
7. Stir in the balsamic vinegar and pesto right into the soup. You can add additional pesto on top if desired. Taste and season as needed.
8. Pesto being drizzled on top of soup.

Prep Time: 5 Minutes

Cook Time: 30 Minutes

Servings: 8

Ingredients

- 1 cup quinoa
- 2 cups water
- 1 tsp salt
- 19 oz canned lentils, drained and rinsed
- 3 tbsp. fresh lemon juice (or more)
- 1 garlic clove, minced
- 2 tbsp. olive oil
- 1 Pepper to taste
- 1 English cucumber, diced
- 2 cups cherry tomatoes, halved
- 2/3 cup parsley, chopped
- 1/2 cup mint, chopped
- 4 scallions, thinly sliced

Instructions

1. Place the quinoa in a medium pot with 2 cups of water and 1 tsp. salt. Bring to a boil, then cover and reduce the heat to medium-low. Cook for 10-15 minutes until the quinoa is fluffy. Drain any excess water if needed. Remove from heat. If you want a cold salad, spread out on a baking sheet to cool or make in advance.
2. Quinoa cooking in a pot on an induction burner.

3. Whisk together the lemon juice, olive oil, garlic, salt, and a few turns of freshly ground black pepper.
4. Olive oil, lemon juice, garlic, and pepper being whisked in a bowl.
5. Toss with quinoa and lentils. Add remaining ingredients and toss together.
6. Wooden tongs tossing together quinoa tabbouleh with lentils.

Prep Time: 15 Minutes

Cook Time: 30 Minutes

Servings: 4

Ingredients

- 20 oz can chickpeas, rinsed and drained
- 3 cups cauliflower florets
- 2 tbsp olive oil
- 2 tsp cumin
- 2 tsp garlic powder
- 1 tsp paprika
- 1 tsp onion powder
- 1 tsp salt
- 1 tsp black pepper
- 1/2 tsp coriander
- 1/4 tsp cinnamon
- 1/16 tsp cayenne
- 8 cups Romaine lettuce
- 1 English cucumber, chopped
- 2 cups cherry tomatoes, chopped
- 1/2 red onion, chopped
- 1/2 cup parsley, chopped
- 1/2 cup hummus

Instructions

1. Preheat the oven to 400 degrees. Make sure the chickpeas are nice and dry. Toss the chickpeas and cauliflower with the olive oil and spices.
2. Chickpeas and cauliflower in a bowl with shawarma spices and olive oil.
3. Lay out flat in a single layer on a baking sheet. Bake for 20-25 minutes until crispy on the outside.
4. Sheet pan with shawarma chickpeas and cauliflower.
5. To serve: Serve over a bed of chopped Romaine lettuce with diced cucumbers, tomatoes, red onions, parsley, and a dollop or drizzle of hummus, tzatziki, or tahini. Pita can be served on the side.
6. Vegan shawarma bowls with chickpeas, cauliflower, tomatoes, cucumber, red onion, and hummus.

Prep Time: 15 Minutes

Cook Time: 45 Minutes

Servings: 6

Ingredients

- 6 fresh beets
- 1/4 cup olive oil
- 2 tbsp balsamic vinegar
- 2 tsp honey (more to taste)
- 2 tsp Dijon mustard (or whole grain mustard)
- Salt and pepper
- 6 cups arugula
- 1 pear, sliced (or apple)
- 1/2 cup goat cheese, crumbled
- 1/4 cup walnuts, chopped

Instructions

1. Preheat the oven to 400 degrees. Scrub the beets well and remove the tops. Wrap each beet in aluminum foil and place it on a baking sheet. Bake for 45-60 minutes (depending on size) until you can easily insert a knife. Let cool until easy to handle. You can also use canned beets or refrigerated cooked beets for a quicker option.
2. Beets being chopped on a cutting board.
3. Peel the beets and then cut them into bite-sized pieces. One easy way to do this is under running water. Just peel the skin back with your hands.

4. Sliced roasted beets on a wooden cutting board.
5. Make the vinaigrette: Whisk together the olive oil, balsamic vinegar, honey, mustard, salt, and pepper.
6. Balsamic vinegar, honey, mustard, olive oil, salt, and pepper in a small dish with a spoon.
7. Assemble the salad with the arugula, beets, pears, walnuts, and goat cheese. Drizzle with vinaigrette. Season with salt and pepper as needed.
8. Goat cheese being sprinkled on a beet and arugula salad with pears.

Prep Time: 10 Minutes

Cook Time: 25 Minutes

Servings: 8

Ingredients

- 10 oz firm tofu, drained well
- 8 rice paper spring roll wrappers
- 1 carrot, thinly sliced
- 1 cucumber, thinly sliced
- 1 cup lettuce
- 1 cup red cabbage, shredded
- 1/8 cup fresh cilantro
- 1/8 cup basil
- 1/8 cup mint
- 1/4 cup peanut butter (or PB2 combined with water)
- 1.5 tbsp low sodium soy sauce
- 1 tbsp pure maple syrup
- 1/2 tbsp fresh lime juice
- 1/2 tbsp rice vinegar
- 1 tsp Asian garlic chili paste (sambal olek)
- 1/8 tsp ground ginger
- 2 tbsp warm water

Instructions

1. To make peanut sauce: Warm the peanut butter in the microwave until slightly melted. This step can be skipped but makes it a bit easier to stir. Add the soy

sauce, maple syrup, lime juice, rice vinegar, garlic chili paste, and ground ginger to a small bowl. Whisk together, adding water a little at a time until it reaches a smooth consistency. It should be thick but still pourable. Taste and adjust seasoning as needed - more soy sauce for salt, more lime juice for tang, more chili paste for heat, etc.

2. Peanut sauce being stirred in a small white bowl.
3. To make the spring rolls, submerge one piece of rice paper into water for 15-20 seconds. Remove and place on a damp cloth. Place the tofu in the center of the paper.
4. Tofu being added to a spring roll wrapper.
5. Layer on the vegetables and herbs. Make sure not to overfill the spring roll or it will break as you are rolling it.
6. Lettuce, carrots, red cabbage, mint, cilantro, and basil being layered on a spring roll wrapper.
7. Carefully fold over one end and then fold over the sides. Then roll over carefully to close the spring roll. Normally there are directions on the rice paper package for rolling.
8. Spring roll being folded and rolled.
9. Serve the spring rolls with the peanut sauce.
10. Fresh spring rolls being drizzled with peanut sauce.

Prep Time: 10 Minutes

Cook Time: 25 Minutes

Servings: 6

Ingredients

- 1 cup brown rice
- 1/4 cup soy sauce (GF if needed)
- 2 tbsp. brown sugar
- 2 tsp. sesame oil
- 3 cloves garlic, minced
- 1 tsp. ginger
- 1/2 tsp. red pepper flakes
- 2 green onions, thinly sliced
- 1 lb. 95% lean ground beef
- 1 cup cabbage, shredded
- 1 cucumber, sliced thin
- 1 red pepper, sliced thin
- 1 cup carrots, shredded
- 1/4 cup cilantro

Instructions

1. Cook the brown rice according to package directions. Prep the vegetables. Normally I like to serve bulgogi with raw vegetables but you could also quickly saute the vegetables if you prefer them cooked.
2. Brown rice being poured into a bowl.
3. Stir together the soy sauce, brown sugar, sesame oil, ginger, garlic, red pepper flakes, and green onions.

4. Green onions being stirred into a bowl or Korean bulgogi sauce.
5. Heat a skillet over medium high heat. Add the beef and brown for 4-6 minutes, breaking up as you go. Add the soy sauce mixture and simmer for 3-4 minutes. Serve over rice with vegetables.
6. Ground beef being stirred in a skillet with Bulgogi sauce.
7. Serve over rice with vegetables. If desired, add some fresh cilantro, a fried egg, and kimchi.
8. Cilantro being added to a bowl with bulgogi ground beef and vegetables.

21. Asian Peanut Slaw

Prep Time: 10 Minutes

Cook Time: 5 Minutes

Servings: 8

Ingredients

- 4 cups cole slaw mix (red and green cabbage and shredded carrots)
- 1 red bell pepper, sliced
- 1 cup shelled edamame
- 1/2 cup jicama, diced
- 3 green onions, chopped
- 1/4 cup chopped cilantro
- 2 tbsp peanuts, chopped (for garnish)
- 1/4 cup peanut butter (or PB2 combined with water)
- 2 tbsp low sodium soy sauce
- 1 tbsp pure maple syrup
- 1 1/2 tsp fresh lime juice
- 1 1/2 tsp rice vinegar
- 1 tsp Asian garlic chili paste
- 1/8 tsp ground ginger
- 1.5 tbsp warm water (more if needed)

Instructions

1. Making the dressing: Warm the peanut butter in the microwave until slightly melted. This step can be skipped but makes it a bit easier to stir. Add the soy

sauce, maple syrup, lime juice, rice vinegar, garlic chili paste, and ground ginger to a small bowl. Whisk together, adding water a little at a time until it reaches a smooth consistency. It should be thick but still pourable. Taste and adjust seasoning as needed - more soy sauce for salt, more lime juice for tang, more chili paste for heat, etc.

2. Peanut butter, soy sauce, maple syrup, lime juice, rice vinegar, and ginger in a bowl.
3. In a large bowl, mix together all of the ingredients. Add the dressing. Mix well and enjoy. I like to let it sit for at least 15 minutes for the flavors to combine.
4. Cabbage slaw, carrots, edamame, cilantro, jicama, and peanut dressing in a bowl.

Prep Time: 10 Minutes

Cook Time: 45 Minutes

Servings: 6

Ingredients

- 2 tsp olive oil
- 4 garlic cloves, minced
- 8 cups spinach
- 2 cup mushrooms, sliced
- 1 zucchini, chopped
- 1.5 cups part skim ricotta cheese
- 1 egg
- 1/4 cup Parmesan cheese
- 1.5 tsp Italian seasoning
- 1 tsp salt
- 1 tsp pepper
- 28 oz canned tomato sauce
- 12 no boil lasagna noodles
- 1 cup shredded part skim mozzarella

Instructions

1. Heat the olive oil in a skillet over medium heat. Add the garlic, spinach, zucchini, and mushrooms. Cook for 5 minute, stirring occasionally. Drain out any excess moisture.
2. In a bowl, mix together the ricotta cheese, egg, Parmesan cheese, salt, pepper, and Italian seasoning. You could also add some red pepper flakes. Set aside.

3. Cover the bottom of the skillet with a thin layer of spaghetti sauce. Add one third of the lasagna noodles to the bottom of the skillet, breaking them up as needed. Then cover with one third of the veggies and ricotta cheese mixture. You can spread it out with a spoon or just add dollops of the cheese. Sprinkle with one third of the mozzarella. Cover with one third of sauce. Repeat to create three layers.
4. Cover and cook on medium low for 20-25 minutes.
5. If desired, place in the oven under the broiler to brown the cheese.

23. Albondigas Soup (Mexican Meatball Soup)

Prep Time: 15 Minutes

Cook Time: 35 Minutes

Servings: 6

Ingredients

- 1.5 lbs 95% lean ground beef (meatballs)
- 1 egg (meatballs)
- 1 cup yellow onion, minced (meatballs)
- 1/4 cup uncooked white rice (Jasmine, for meatballs)
- 3 garlic cloves, minced (soup)
- 2 tbsp fresh mint, minced (meatballs, optional)
- 2 tbsp fresh cilantro, chopped (meatballs)
- 1 tsp kosher salt (meatballs)
- 1/2 tsp oregano (meatballs)
- 1/2 tsp cumin (meatballs)
- 1/2 tsp black pepper (meatballs)
- 1 tbsp olive oil (soup)
- 1 onion, diced (soup)
- 2 carrots, peeled and chopped (soup)
- 2 celery stalks, chopped (soup)
- 2 jalapeno peppers, minced (seeds and veins removed, for soup)
- 1 large potato, chopped (soup)
- 3 tbsp tomato paste (soup)
- 5 cups chicken broth (soup)
- 1 cup canned tomato sauce (soup)
- 1 bay leaf (soup)
- 2 small zucchini, chopped (soup)
- 1 cup corn (fresh or frozen, for soup)

Instructions

1. Meatballs: Combine the ground beef, egg, onion, white rice, garlic, mint, cilantro, salt, oregano, cumin, and black pepper in a large bowl. Gently mix together with your hands until combined. Use a rounded tablespoon to roll the mixture into meatballs. Refrigerate until ready to use.
2. Albondigas made with ground beef, white rice, and herbs rolled on a plate.
3. Heat the olive oil over medium high heat in a large soup pot or Dutch oven. Add the onion, carrots, celery, jalapenos, and potato. Cook for 5-7 minutes until beginning to soften. Add the garlic and tomato paste. Cook for 1-2 minutes until the garlic is fragrant.
4. Carrots, onions, jalapeños, celery, and jalapenos cooking in a soup pot.
5. Add the chicken broth and tomato sauce. Bring to a simmer. Season well with salt and pepper.
6. Tomato sauce and chicken broth being added to a soup pot with vegetables.
7. Add the meatballs and cover. Cook for 30 minutes without stirring. Stirring can break the meatballs.
8. Mexican meatballs simmering in a pot with tomato broth.
9. Open and add the zucchini and corn. Cook for 5-10 minutes longer until the meatballs are cooked through and the rice is tender. Serve with cilantro, fresh limes, radishes, etc.
10. Albondigas soup served in a white bowl with cilantro and radishes.

Prep Time: 10 Minutes

Cook Time: 25 Minutes

Servings: 4

Ingredients

- 1 tbsp. olive oil
- 1 lb 99% lean ground turkey
- 2 garlic cloves, minced
- 1/2 onion, chopped
- 1 red pepper, diced
- 2 cups butternut squash, peeled and chopped
- 1 cup canned diced tomatoes (not drained)
- Salt and pepper
- 1 tsp. Italian seasoning
- 1/4 tsp. red pepper flakes
- 1 cup reduced fat feta cheese (or mozzarella)

Instructions

1. Heat the olive oil in a skillet over medium high heat. Add the turkey and cook, breaking up the meat, for 6-8 minutes. Add the garlic, onion, and red bell pepper. Cook for 4-5 minutes until the onion begins to brown.
2. Ground turkey, diced onions, and diced bell pepper in a skillet.
3. Add the butternut squash, tomatoes, salt, pepper, Italian seasoning, and red pepper flakes. Cover the skillet and cook until the butternut squash is tender, about 6-8 minutes. Add a touch of water or broth if

anything begins to burn. Depending on the size of the butternut squash, it could take a bit longer. For quick-cooking preparation, make sure to cut it into small pieces.
4. Ground turkey, butternut squash, tomatoes in a skillet with Italian seasoning being added.
5. Add the cheese and cover for 1-2 minutes until it melts.
6. Ground turkey with butternut squash and tomatoes in a bowl topped with feta cheese.

Prep Time: 15 Minutes

Cook Time: 15 Minutes

Servings: 4

Ingredients

- 1.33 lbs boneless skinless chicken breast
- Salt and pepper
- 1 tbsp olive oil
- 1 tbsp fresh rosemary, minced (leaves only)
- 2 garlic cloves, minced
- 1/4 cup low sodium chicken broth
- 2 tbsp lemon juice
- 2 tsp honey (optional)
- 1 tbsp melted butter

Instructions

1. Preheat the oven to 400 degrees. Season the chicken with salt and pepper. Make sure the chicken breasts are a similar thickness, if needed slightly pound the chicken in the thickest part.
2. Chicken breast being seasoned with salt and pepper.
3. In a small bowl. combine the rosemary, garlic, chicken broth, lemon juice, melted butter, and honey.
4. Garlic, rosemary, honey, lemon juice, and chicken broth being stirred together in a bowl.
5. Heat the olive oil over medium-high in a heavy, oven are skillet. Sear the chicken for 2-3 minutes on each side, until browned.

6. Chicken breast searing in a pan.
7. Pour the sauce over the chicken. Place the skillet in the oven. Cook for 14-18 minutes (depending on thickness) until the chicken reaches 165 degrees. Halfway through cooking, open the oven and baste the chicken with sauce. Serve with extra lemon slices.
8. Chicken being cooked in a rosemary pan sauce in a cast iron skillet.

Prep Time: 15 Minutes

Cook Time: 4hrs 15 Minutes

Servings: 4

Ingredients

- 2 tbsp olive oil
- 4 cups eggplant, cubed
- 2 zucchini, cubed
- 1 summer squash, chopped
- 2 bell peppers, chopped
- 1 cup red onion, sliced
- 1.5 cups mushrooms
- 4 garlic cloves, minced
- 1 tbsp Italian seasoning
- 28 oz can fire roasted diced tomatoes
- Salt and pepper
- 2 tbsp balsamic vinegar
- 18 oz. prepared polenta tube

Instructions

1. Add the olive oil, eggplant, zucchini, summer squash, bell peppers, onion, mushroom, garlic, Italian seasoning, tomatoes, salt, and pepper to the slow cooker. For a more traditional ratatouille layer the vegetables.
2. Vegetables and herbs being added to a slow cooker for ratatouille.

3. Cook on low for 4 hours. When ready to serve, stir in the balsamic vinegar and fresh herbs if desired.
4. Ratatouille in a bowl being topped with fresh herbs and vinegar.
5. To make the polenta rounds, preheat the oven to 400 degrees and slice the polenta in 3/4 inch rounds. Season with salt and pepper. Place on a prepared baking sheet and cook for 10 minutes, flipping halfway through.
6. Polenta rounds baking in the oven with olive oil, salt, and pepper.

Prep Time: 15 Minutes

Cook Time: 15 Minutes

Servings: 4

Ingredients

- 1.5 lbs. boneless skinless chicken breast
- 1 tbsp. olive oil
- 1 tsp. cumin
- 1 tsp garlic powder
- 1/2 tsp. paprika
- 1/2 tsp. kosher salt
- 1/4 tsp. black pepper
- 1/4 tsp. red pepper flakes (optional)
- 1 lime (or lemon, for serving)

Instructions

1. Preheat the grill or grill pan over medium-high heat. Mix together the cumin, garlic powder, paprika, salt, pepper, and red pepper flakes in a small bowl.
2. Cumin, paprika, garlic powder, kosher salt, pepper, and red chili flakes in a small bowl.
3. Brush the chicken breasts with olive oil. Sprinkle over the chicken and rub it in to evenly coat the chicken.
4. Chicken breast being coated with a cumin seasoning rub.
5. Grill for 4-6 minutes per side or until cooked through. Tent with foil and let rest for 5 minutes. Serve with freshly squeezed lime juice.

6. Cumin chicken breasts grilling on a grill pan.

Prep Time: 10 Minutes

Cook Time: 15 Minutes

Servings: 4

Ingredients

- 1.5 lbs cod (thick cut filets, 4 filets)
- 1/3 cup flour
- 3/4 tsp sweet paprika
- 3/4 tsp Italian seasoning
- 3/4 tsp kosher salt
- 1/2 tsp cumin
- 1/2 tsp fresh ground black pepper
- 1 tbsp olive oil (more if needed)
- 1 tbsp butter

Instructions

1. Pat the fish dry using paper towels.
2. Cod fish filets on a plate with flour on the side.
3. In a shallow dish, combine the flour, sweet paprika, Italian seasoning, salt, cumin, and pepper. Dredge the fish in the flour on both sides so it is lightly coated.
4. Cod fish being dredged in flour and spices.
5. Heat the olive oil and butter over medium-high heat in a heavy-bottomed skillet. Once the oil is shimmering, add the fish. Cook for 4-6 minutes until the fish is nicely browned and easily releases from the pan. Flip and cook on the other side for 4-6 minutes until cooked through and lightly browned.

6. Cod being pan seared in a hot skillet.

7. Ingredients for 4 servings: 1 tbsp butter, 2-4 garlic
    cloves, 2 tbsp capers (optional), 1/2 cup dry white
    wine (or chicken broth), 1/4 cup chopped parsley.
    Once the fish is cooked, add a drizzle of olive oil to the
    pan. Add the garlic and capers to the pan. Cook for 1
    minute until fragrant. Add the white wine to deglaze
    the pan. Scrape any browned bits from the bottom of
    the pan. Bring to a boil and cook for about 1 minute.
    Stir in the lemon juice and parsley. Serve over fish.

8. White wine pan sauce with capers and garlic in a
    skillet.

Prep Time: 15 Minutes

Cook Time: 20Minutes

Servings: 8

Ingredients

- 2 tbsp olive oil (for grilled vegetables)
- 2 tbsp lemon juice (marinade/dressing)
- 2 tbsp balsamic vinegar (marinade/dressing)
- 1 tbsp Dijon mustard (marinade/dressing)
- 1 tbsp honey (optional, marinade/dressing)
- 2 garlic cloves, minced (marinade/dressing)
- 1 tsp Italian seasoning (marinade/dressing)
- 1/2 tsp kosher salt (marinade/dressing)
- 1/2 tsp black pepper (marinade/dressing)
- 2 zucchini
- 2 bell peppers
- 1 red onion
- 1 lb asparagus
- 2 cups mushrooms, halved
- 8 oz penne pasta (cooked and cooled)
- 1/4 cup parsley, chopped
- 1/4 cup fresh basil, chopped
- 4 oz crumbled feta cheese (or goat cheese)
- Salt and pepper

Instructions

1. Make the dressing/mariande: Add all of the ingredients to a bowl or mason jar. Stir or whisk well to combine. When the vegetables come off the grill, drizzle 2/3 of the dressing over the vegetables. Let rest for 5 minutes. Save the rest of the dressing for serving with the pasta salad.
2. Balsamic vinaigrette in a glass jar.
3. To grill vegetables: Cut the vegetables into larger slices that won't fall through the grill grates, about ½ inch thick. For the zucchini, it is best to cut it on the diagonal. Cut bell peppers into larger slices. Cut the red onion into rings. Trim the asparagus ends. Toss the vegetables with olive oil, salt, and pepper. Start by grilling the red onions, mushrooms, and bell peppers. They will take 3-5 minutes per side. Then add the asparagus and zucchini. It will take 2-4 minutes per side.
4. Asparagus and zucchini on a grill pan.
5. Assemble salad: Chop the vegetables into bite-sized pieces if desired. Toss the grilled vegetables with the pasta and the remaining dressing. Top with feta cheese and fresh herbs.
6. Cooked pasta, feta cheese, fresh herbs, and grilled vegetables in a bowl for pasta salad.

Prep Time: 15 Minutes

Cook Time: 20 Minutes

Servings: 4

Ingredients

- 1 lb lean beef tenderloin (or other tender steak)
- 2 tbsp blackening seasoning
- 1 tsp lime zest
- 1 tbsp butter (or ghee or olive oil)
- 2 tsp grapeseed oil (or olive or vegetable)
- 8 small flour tortillas (small)
- 1 cup salsa (pineapple salsa below)
- 1/4 cup cilantro

Instructions

1. Preheat the oven to 375. Let the steak come to room temp. Heat a cast-iron skillet over medium-high heat for 5 minutes. Meanwhile, rub butter over both sides of the steak. Generously rub steak with seasoning. If needed, cut the steak into chunks so it will fit in the pan.
2. Steak covered in blackening seasoning on a cutting boad.
3. Add the grapeseed oil to the skillet. Substitute olive oil if no grapeseed oil is available, I like to use grapeseed oil for its high smoke point. Just make sure to have the exhaust fan on high. Place steak into the cast iron

skillet and cook for 2 minutes per side. Turn off the heat.

4. Steak being blackened in a cast iron skillet.
5. Place cast iron into the oven for 5 minutes for rare, 6 minutes for medium rare, or 7 minutes for medium. Check temp with a meat thermometer, Steak will rise 5 degrees as it rests. (Remove at 120* for rare, 130* for medium rare, and 140* for medium). Remove from the oven and place on a cutting board. Let rest for 5 minutes. Slice steak into strips.
6. Sliced blackened steak on a cutting board.
7. While the steak rests, warm the tortillas and prep any taco toppings.
8. Slcied blackened steak with flour tortillas, cheese, and jalapenos for tacos.